Yohimbe

(*Pausinystalia johimbe*)

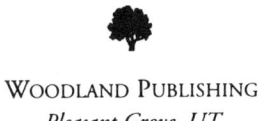

WOODLAND PUBLISHING
Pleasant Grove, UT

© 1997
Woodland Publishing, Inc.
P.O. Box 160
Pleasant Grove, UT
84062

Contents

YOHIMBE — AN INTRODUCTION   5

PRIMARY APPLICATIONS OF YOHIMBE   7

RECENT YOHIMBE STUDIES   12

CONCLUSION   13

ENDNOTES   15

Yohimbe

(Pausinystalia johimbe)

Yohimbe – An Introduction

Yohimbe has become a popular herbal remedy for the treatment of male sexual dysfunction. It is considered to be one of the few natural aphrodisiacs. Its stimulatory and aphrodisiacal effects have been studied and documented. Research is ongoing as to the use of yohimbe for impotence and other disorders. Studies have shown that the use of yohimbe specifically increases the blood flow in the genital regions of both males and females. Results have been positive in treating male impotence, and studies continue to validate its use for this condition. Yohimbe is known to dilate blood vessels near the skin, mucous membranes and sex organs to help with various disorders and improved sexual function.

The yohimbe tree grows wild along the tropical west coast of Africa from Nigeria to Gabon. It is a tall evergreen with large, leathery leaves. The inner bark has been used traditionally to treat angina and hypertension. It was also smoked and snuffed by natives for its hallucinogenic effect.[1] In some areas of western Africa including Ghana, the Ivory Coast and Upper Volta, a decoction is used to treat fevers and leprosy. It is also chewed to help relieve a cough.[2]

Yohimbe bark was first brought to the attention of Europeans by early traders. While on expeditions in western Africa, they heard stories about the yohimbe tree. Traders became interested in discovering and experiencing the legendary yohimbe bark. When they returned to Europe with the yohimbe bark and tales of its "powers," European interest in and demand for the bark began to grow.

YOHIMBE'S HISTORY

Yohimbe has long been used for its aphrodisiac effects. In West Africa, yohimbe bark has long been valued as an aphrodisiac. For centuries many native people of West Africa have made a tea from the bark. The tea treats impotence and works as a sexual stimulant. The folklore surrounding yohimbe's use as an aphrodisiac is considerable. In the past, the yohimbe bark was rubbed on the body, smoked, sniffed and ingested to increase sexual desire and performance.[3] Europeans were very interested in the bark of the yohimbe tree when they heard about it from the natives. Since those first trips to western Africa, people throughout the world have looked for the valued yohimbe bark.

There are only a few herbs available that are considered to be aphrodisiacs. Generally, these herbs are taken only occasionally to increase stimulation, sexual pleasure and sexual performance. Yohimbe is sometimes found in combination with other herbs such as damiana, muira puama, ginseng and saw palmetto.

YOHIMBINE

Yohimbine is the active ingredient found in the yohimbe bark. Both the crude bark and the purified compound are used as aphrodisiacs.[4] The yohimbine content is thought to be approximately 6 percent. Other minor alkaloids found in yohimbe bark include ajmaline, alloyohimbine, corynanthine, quebrachine and tetrahydromethylcorynanthein.[5] Compounds found in yohimbe are known to be a precursor of testosterone.

Yohimbine is the only medicine approved for treating erectile dysfunction.[6] It is listed in the *Physicians Desk Reference* as a sensual stimulant. Yohimbine aids the increase of sexual desire, but its main function is to increase the blood flow to the erectile tissue.[7] It has been found to be effective in treating both organic (physiological) and psychogenic (mental) forms of impotence.

Primary Applications of Yohimbe

IMPOTENCE

Impotence is defined as the inability to achieve and maintain a penile erection. It is the most common sexual disorder among men. It is estimated that 10 to 20 million men suffer from some form of erectile dysfunction and it is estimated that 25 percent of men over the age of 50 suffer from some form of impotence. Also new cases are on the rise as the median age of the population increases. The prevalence of impotence rises with age, though this is not thought to be the main reason for the problem. It is true that the physical need to ejaculate and the force of the ejaculation do decrease with age. Most men are thought to be able to retain an erection well into their 80s.[8] Approximately half of the population of men are considered impotent by the age of 75. Aging is a factor in impotence, due in part to lower levels of testosterone and poor circulation caused by atherosclerosis.

Men suffering from impotence may have feelings of humiliation, worthlessness and despair. It can lead to depression in some individuals. Many feel that their sex life is over and may even stop trying. However, in many cases impotence is reversible and temporary. Yohimbe may be a remedy that can help individuals suffering from impotence.

Most cases of impotence are organic in nature. It used to be thought by most professionals that the cause was generally due to psychological disorders. Men were told to relax and reduce stress in their lives to help in resuming sexual function. This is no longer the case. Today this condition is recognized by most doctors as being physiologically based. Impotence can result from various organic problems such as atherosclerosis, diabetes, Parkinson's disease, kidney disease, stroke, epilepsy, endocrine disorders, hypothyroidism, male sexual organ problems, vascular insufficiency or drug, alcohol and tobacco use. Of course, along with physiological problems, there are still psychogenic problems involving impotence which are usually caused by depression, tension, anxiety and stress.

Atherosclerosis is thought to be the most frequent cause of impotence. An erection occurs as the nerve impulses cause the dilation of the arteries of the penis. This allows blood to build up in the erectile tissue. When atherosclerosis is a problem, the blood vessels are not able to supply sufficient blood to achieve an erection.

The important thing to remember is that there are ways to deal with impotence. A thorough medical exam may help evaluate and understand the cause. Natural methods, such as the use of yohimbe, may also be useful in treating impotence. It is important to be in contact with a medical professional when trying any method of treatment for impotence.

Blood Vessel Dilation

Yohimbine, the active component found in yohimbe, is well known for its ability to dilate blood vessels and lower blood pressure. It dilates the vessels of the skin and mucous membranes. The aphrodisiac effects associated with yohimbe are related to this dilation. Yohimbe increases the blood flow and enlarges the vessels in the sexual organs as well as increases reflex excitability in the lower spinal cord.[9] Yohimbe has been found to make the erections harder and firmer through the increased circulation to the area. It is also thought to aid in maintaining an erection by causing a compression and preventing the blood from flowing out of the organ.

Poor circulation is known to be one cause of impotence and erectile dysfunction. Vascular disease is known to be a major factor in many cases of impotence. Atherosclerosis in the body also effects the penile artery reducing circulation to that area. Atherosclerosis is a common cause of impotence.[10] Reducing cardiovascular risk factors can help reduce the incidence of impotence. Obesity, smoking, high blood pressure, and elevated cholesterol can increase problems of impotence. Yohimbe can help through increasing the vessel dilation and improving circulation to the sexual organs in the body.

Sexual Dysfunction

Yohimbe has become popular as an aphrodisiac for both men and women. Yohimbine hydrochloride is found in some prescription drugs for the treatment of male impotence.[11] A study done using rats in 1984 gave small doses of yohimbine to sexually active male rats. Though they showed normal sexual activity before, their sexual arousal increased with the addition of the yohimbine.[12] It seems to have a similar effect in humans. This has lead to an increase in studies involving yohimbe and yohimbine.

Yohimbe stimulates reactions in the body to aid some cases of impotence, due to fatigue, tension, and stress. Yohimbe is found to be useful in increasing blood flow to the corpus cavernosom to aid in increasing the strength and length of the erection of the penis. It may also help to increase the production of norepinephrine in the body, which is known to decrease with age, and effects the formation of erections. The adrenaline supply may also increase which can heighten the male sensual stimulation.[13]

YOHIMBE AND THE CENTRAL NERVOUS SYSTEM

Evidence points to yohimbe as a central nervous system stimulant. The alkaloid yohimbine was found to stimulate the respiratory center when taken in small doses. In large doses, it was found to actually depress respiration. It easily penetrates the central nervous system causing a variety of responses. Some of the responses include excitation, elevated blood pressure, increased heart rate and increased motor activity in animals and humans.[14]

YOHIMBE AND HORMONAL PRODUCTION

As we age, the body's hormonal system slows down. This can lead to problems with sexual dysfunction. Yohimbe is thought to help suppress the action often associated with a decrease in production of certain hormones due to the aging process. Yohimbe is considered an alpha-adrenoreceptor blocker. Such a blocker possesses the ability to reduce the effects of hormones that increase the constriction of blood vessels with age. It also increases the body's production of norepinephrine which is important for erections. Yohimbe has also been found to increase the adrenaline reaching the nerve endings to stimulate sensations and allow for a more fulfilling sexual experience. Yohimbe may help to rejuvenate the male libido and restore normal sexual function due to a slowing down of the hormonal system that often accompanies aging.

YOHIMBE AND EXERCISE

Yohimbe is found in some herbal formulas used for endurance, sustained strength during exercise and for body building. This reaction is thought to be due to yohimbe being a precursor to testosterone. Increased testosterone levels are believed to improve strength and endurance. The stimulation of certain hormones, such as testosterone, seems to help with athletic performance.[15] Many professional athletes look for methods of improving their performance and have found beneficial results using yohimbe.

YOHIMBE AND FATIGUE IN AIDS PATIENTS

Yohimbine, the active ingredient found in yohimbe bark, has been used by a few AIDS patients for treating fatigue. These patients' physicians had no anticipation of yohimbine being useful in helping with fatigue. Very little, if any, long-term clinical studies have been done on yohimbine with regard to treating fatigue. The patients using yohimbine felt much better and showed a definite improvement in quality of life. The individuals taking the yohimbe were very impressed with their results. It is important to remember that most AIDS patients are taking medications and yohimbine should only be used under the care of a medical professional for AIDS.[16]

Recent Yohimbe Studies

CANADIAN STUDY

Alvaro Morales, a urologist at Queen's University in Kingston, Ontario, Canada, has conducted a study using yohimbine, the active component found in the yohimbe bark. Some physical conditions can lead to impotence due primarily to decreased circulation and vascular problems. Twenty-three men with problems of physical impotence from conditions such as diabetes and heart disease were given yohimbine daily for eight to ten weeks. Ten of the men improved and six were able to sustain an erection and reach orgasm. One other interesting note is the fact that many of the men had less prickling and numbness in their legs which is often associated with diabetes. This could be accounted for by the improved vascular dilation and circulation that resulted when using yohimbine. Side effects were mild; most common were temporary dizziness and gastrointestinal upset. This same team of researchers is now conducting a two year long study involving 120 men with impotence from organic or psychological origin.[17]

ITALIAN STUDY

An Italian clinical study was conducted in 1994 using yohimbine for cases of impotence. The individuals involved in the study were suffering from psychogenic forms of impotence due to stress, tension and fatigue. Half of the patients received yohimbe tablets and the other half a placebo. The study continued for eight weeks. The group taking the yohimbe had a 71 percent success rate while the placebo group had only a 22 percent improvement. The placebo group then had the opportunity of trying the yohimbe tablets and the positive results reached 74 percent among the placebo group. The study also found that yohimbe had the ability of stimulating the male libido.[18] The men were generally more aroused and interested in sexual experiences. Though the increased arousal has not been fully documented, many individuals have claimed to be sexually stimulated while taking yohimbe.

AMERICAN STUDY

A recent study published in the *Journal of Urology* tested yohimbine on a group of men who suffered from chronic sexual dysfunction. The men all took a moderate dose of yohimbine for one month. The improvement rate for men who had suffered impotence for less than two years was 81 percent. These results are very encouraging as the improvement was seen quickly. There was also significant improvement for men who had trouble sustaining an erection. They reported fuller and more lasting erections.[19] The results for all the studies have been positive.

Conclusion

The herb yohimbe has been recognized by many people from many different cultures as an effective way to deal with forms of sexual impotence, as well as fatigue and effects of aging. Used correctly, yohimbe can enhance the quality of one's life.

SAFETY

Some medical professionals feel that yohimbe should be avoided because of the possible side effects associated with its use. The use of yohimbe should be closely watched and monitored for side effects. Yohimbine is thought to be toxic if ingested in high doses.[20] It may induce panic attacks, hallucinations, elevated blood pressure, increased heart rate, dizziness, and headaches. It is not recommended for individuals suffering from heart conditions, kidney disease, psychological problems or women.[21] Yohimbine may lead to psychoses in individuals with a predisposition.[22] Overuse may lead to fatigue, stomach disorders or weakness.[23] If an individual's blood pressure is normally low, yohimbe may cause fatigue and even temporary impotence.[24]

Yohimbe should not be used in combination or at the same time as food containing tyramine, an amino acid. Foods high in tyramine include cheese, liver, and red wine. Diet aids and decongestants containing phenylpropanolamine should also be avoided.[25]

There have been reports of yohimbe products not actually containing yohimbe. Some French and American yohimbine products were analyzed and did not contain any yohimbe, only caffeine.[26] This can be a problem with any herbal or natural health product. Reputable herbal companies regularly analyze their own products before selling to the public.

It is important to note that most, if not all, of the research done has been on the isolated component, yohimbine. Use of the whole yohimbe bark may be wise. Often single components can cause more side effects than using the whole plant. It is thought to be safe when taken in recommended dosages. Medical doctors have prescribed drugs containing yohimbine to thousands of patients with positive results. But it is always prudent to use caution with any drug or herbal remedy.

Availability

Yohimbine is available in prescription combinations under the brand names Yocon™, Yohimex™ and Aphrodyne™. Yohimbe bark extracts are available in health food stores in most states. It is important to follow the recommended dosages and buy from a reputable herbal company to ensure purity and safety. Impurities in some combinations have caused concern by some health professionals. Choose a respected product from a company that uses strict quality control guidelines.

Endnotes

1. The Lawrence Review of Natural Products, May 1993, 1.
2. James Duke, Handbook of Medicinal Herbs, Boca Raton, Florida: CRC Press, Inc. 1985, p 351.
3. Jack Ritchason, The Little Herb Encyclopedia. Pleasant Grove, UT: Woodland Books, 1994, 263.
4. The Lawrence Review of Natural Products, 1.
5. Duke, 351.
6. Michael T. Murray, N.D., Male Sexual Vitality, Rocklin, CA: Prima Publishing, 1994, p 26.
7. Michael T. Murray, N.D., Let's Live, "Sexual Vitality for Men and Women." May 1994, 16.
8. Michael T. Murray, N.D., Let's Live, "Natural Approaches To Impotence." July, 1995, 44.
9. Varro E. Tyler, Ph.D.., The Honest Herbal. New York: Pharmaceutical Products Press, 1993, 327.
10. Michael T. Murray, N.D., Let's Live, "Natural Approaches To

Impotence." July, 1995, 44.

11. Natural Health Handbook, Brookline Village, MA: Boston Common Press Ltd. Partnership, 1995, 75.

12. Tyler, 328.

13. Healthsource Home Page, K2 Consulting Inc., 1996.

14. A. Leung and Steven Foster, Encyclopedia of Common Natural Ingredients Used in Food, Drugs and Cosmetics. 1996, 523.

15. Ritchason, 263.

16. John S. James, AIDS Treatment News, "Yohimbine: Accidental Discovery As Fatigue Treatment?" Sept. 18, 1992, 159.

17. Duke, 351.

18. Healthsource.

19. Ibid.

20. The Lawrence Review of Natural Products, 1.

21. Murray, Male Sexual Vitality., 26.

22. The Lawrence Review of Natural Products, 1.

23. Anna Carr, et. al., Rodale's Illustrated Encyclopedia of Herbs, Emmaus, Pennsylvania: Rodale Press, 1987, 520.

24. Ritchason, 263.

25. Tyler, 328.

26. Quarterly Review of Natural Products., Spring 1995, 31.